DEDICATION

This I ROCKED CANCER TO THE CORE Chemo Journal is dedicated to all those overwhelmed individuals & families out there who are looking to make their journey just a little bit smoother. We know that staying organized and writing out your thoughts and feelings during this time is essential.

YOU are my inspiration for producing this ROCKER Musician Centered Chemo Journal and I'm honored to be a part of keeping all of your essential thoughts, experiences, emotions and notes organized all in one easy to find spot. We're honored and glad if we help make your day easier in any way!

THIS JOURNAL BELONGS TO
_____
_____
_____
_____

DATE _____
CHEMO DRUG _____
DAY# _____ AFTER CHEMO # _____

TODAY I FEEL

_____
_____
_____
_____

EXERCISE **FOOD & DRINK** **SLEEP**
☐ ☐ ☐
☐ ☐ ☐
☐ ☐ ☐

GRATITUDE ◉ ◉ ◉ ◉ ◉ ◉

NOTES
_____
_____
_____
_____
_____
_____
_____
_____
_____
_____

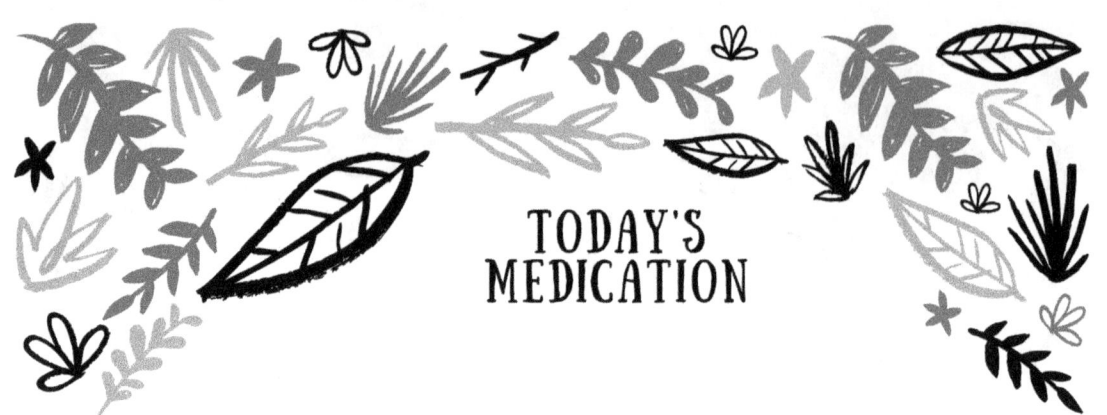

TODAY'S MEDICATION

TIME	MEDICATION	DOSAGE	REACTIONS

DATE _____
CHEMO DRUG _____
DAY # _____ AFTER CHEMO # _____

TODAY I FEEL

_____
_____
_____
_____

EXERCISE **FOOD & DRINK** **SLEEP**
☐ ☐ ☐
☐ ☐ ☐
☐ ☐ ☐

GRATITUDE ⬤⬤⬤⬤⬤⬤

NOTES
_____
_____
_____
_____
_____
_____
_____
_____
_____
_____
_____

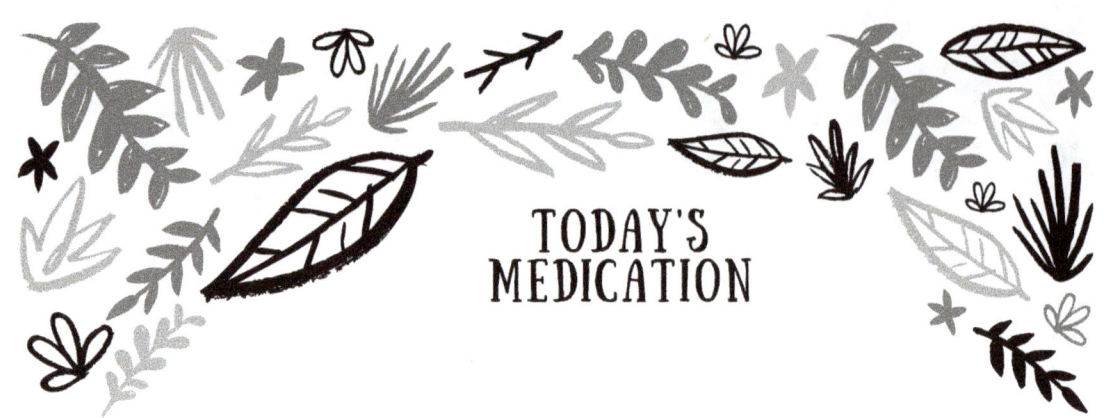

TODAY'S MEDICATION

TIME	MEDICATION	DOSAGE	REACTIONS

DATE _____
CHEMO DRUG _____
DAY # _____ AFTER CHEMO # _____

TODAY I FEEL

_____
_____
_____
_____

EXERCISE
☐
☐
☐

FOOD & DRINK
☐
☐
☐

SLEEP
☐
☐
☐

GRATITUDE

NOTES
_____
_____
_____
_____
_____
_____
_____
_____
_____
_____

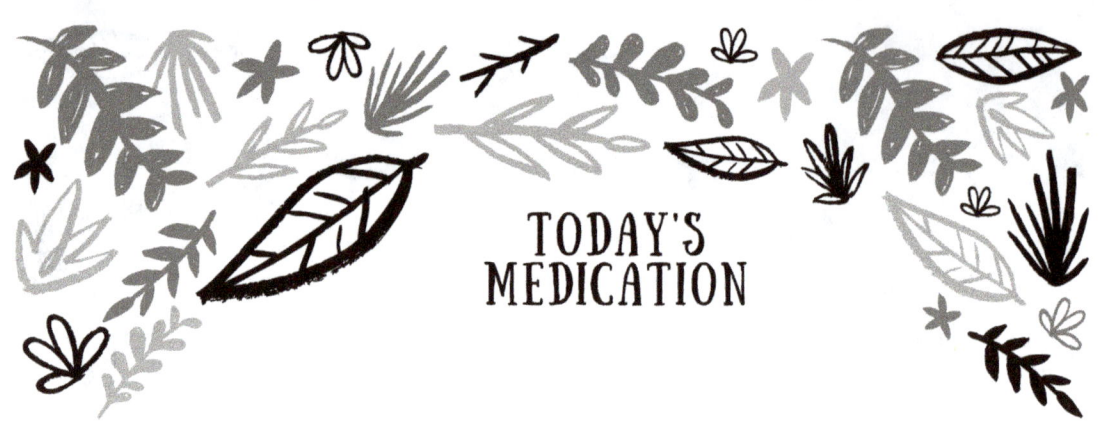

TODAY'S MEDICATION

TIME	MEDICATION	DOSAGE	REACTIONS

DATE _____
CHEMO DRUG _____
DAY # _____ AFTER CHEMO # _____

TODAY I FEEL

_____
_____
_____
_____

EXERCISE
☐
☐
☐

FOOD & DRINK
☐
☐
☐

SLEEP
☐
☐
☐

GRATITUDE

NOTES
_____
_____
_____
_____
_____
_____
_____
_____
_____
_____
_____

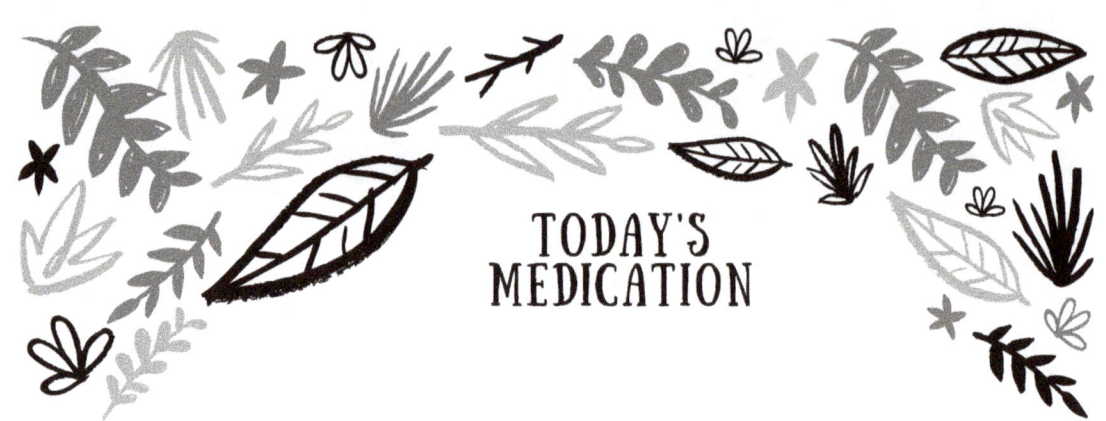

TODAY'S MEDICATION

TIME	MEDICATION	DOSAGE	REACTIONS

DATE _____
CHEMO DRUG _____
DAY# _____ AFTER CHEMO # _____

TODAY I FEEL

_____
_____
_____

EXERCISE **FOOD & DRINK** **SLEEP**
☐ ☐ ☐
☐ ☐ ☐
☐ ☐ ☐

GRATITUDE **NOTES**
_____
_____
_____
_____
_____
_____
_____
_____
_____
_____

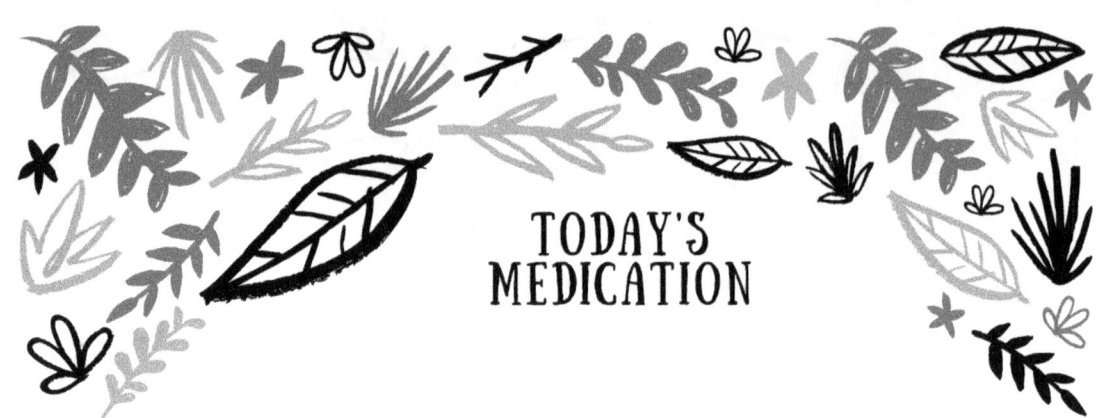

TODAY'S MEDICATION

TIME	MEDICATION	DOSAGE	REACTIONS

DATE _____
CHEMO DRUG _____
DAY # _____ AFTER CHEMO # _____

TODAY I FEEL

_____
_____
_____
_____

EXERCISE **FOOD & DRINK** **SLEEP**

☐ ☐ ☐
☐ ☐ ☐
☐ ☐ ☐

GRATITUDE

⬤ ⬤ ⬤ ⬤ ⬤ ⬤

NOTES

_____
_____
_____
_____
_____
_____
_____
_____
_____
_____

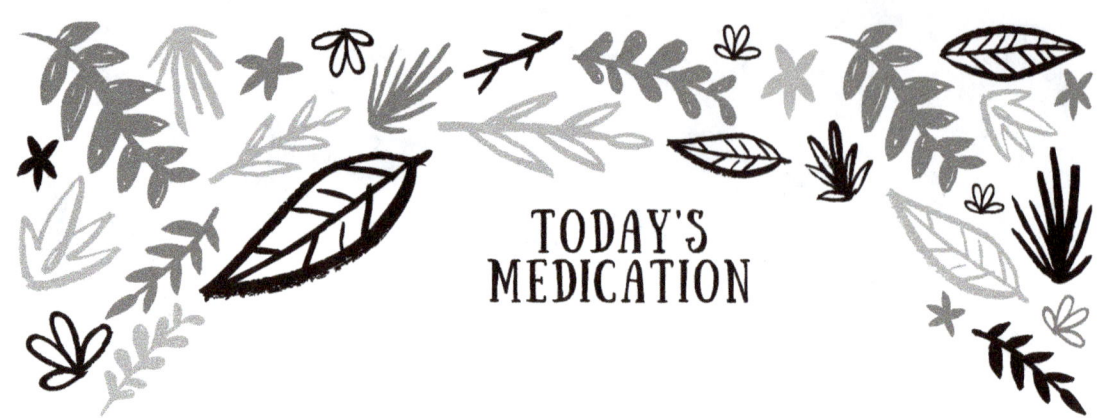

TODAY'S MEDICATION

TIME	MEDICATION	DOSAGE	REACTIONS

DATE _____
CHEMO DRUG _____
DAY# _____ AFTER CHEMO # _____

TODAY I FEEL

_____
_____
_____
_____

EXERCISE
☐
☐
☐

FOOD & DRINK
☐
☐
☐

SLEEP
☐
☐
☐

GRATITUDE

NOTES
_____
_____
_____
_____
_____
_____
_____
_____
_____
_____

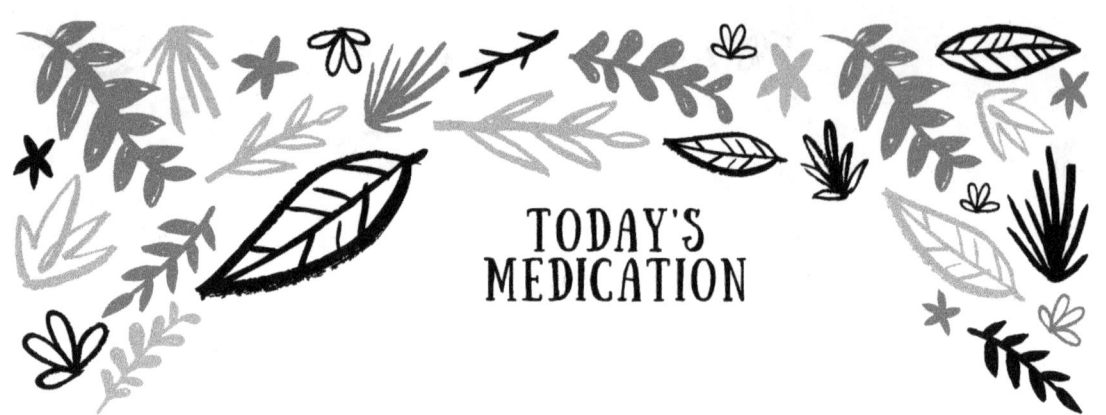

TODAY'S MEDICATION

TIME	MEDICATION	DOSAGE	REACTIONS

DATE _____
CHEMO DRUG _____
DAY# _____ AFTER CHEMO # _____

TODAY I FEEL

_____
_____
_____
_____

EXERCISE   **FOOD & DRINK**   **SLEEP**
☐   ☐   ☐
☐   ☐   ☐
☐   ☐   ☐

GRATITUDE   ⬤ ⬤ ⬤ ⬤ ⬤ ⬤

NOTES
_____
_____
_____
_____
_____
_____
_____
_____
_____
_____

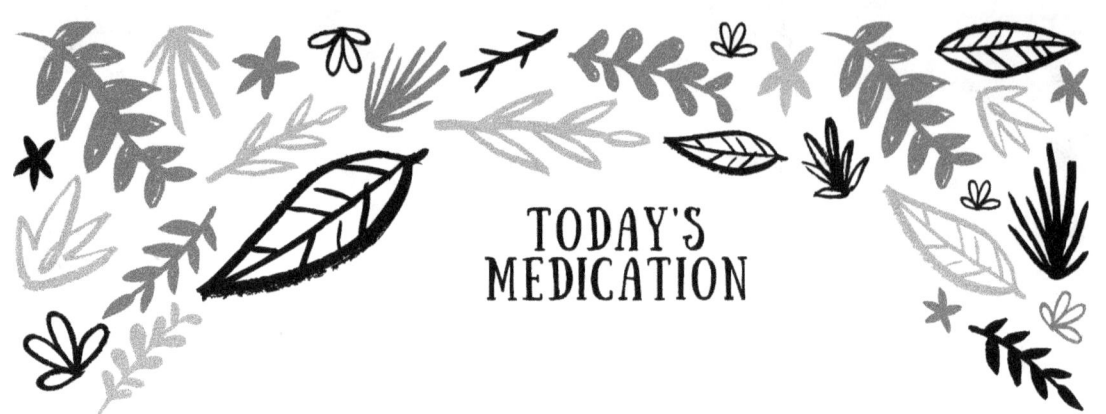

TODAY'S MEDICATION

TIME	MEDICATION	DOSAGE	REACTIONS

DATE _____
CHEMO DRUG _____
DAY # _____ AFTER CHEMO # _____

TODAY I FEEL

_____
_____
_____

EXERCISE
☐
☐
☐

FOOD & DRINK
☐
☐
☐

SLEEP
☐
☐
☐

GRATITUDE

NOTES

_____
_____
_____
_____
_____
_____
_____
_____
_____
_____

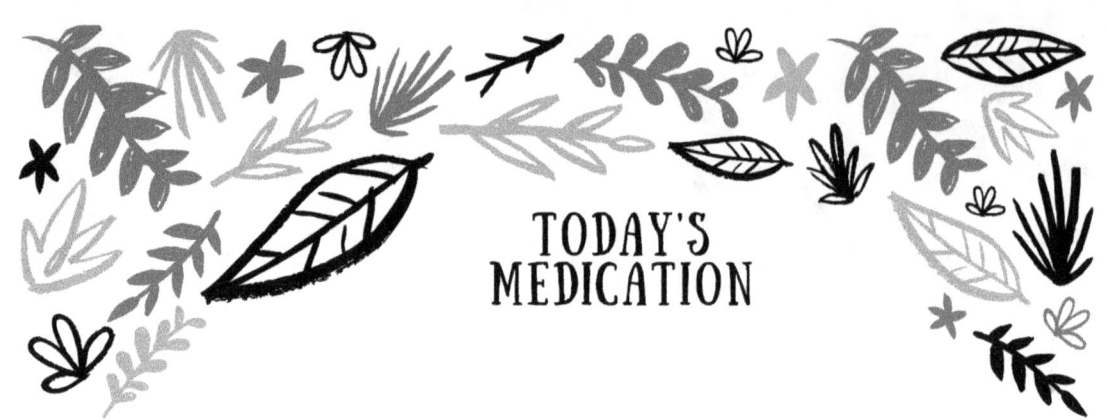

TODAY'S MEDICATION

TIME	MEDICATION	DOSAGE	REACTIONS

DATE _____
CHEMO DRUG _____
DAY # _____ AFTER CHEMO # _____

TODAY I FEEL

_____
_____
_____
_____

EXERCISE **FOOD & DRINK** **SLEEP**
☐ ☐ ☐
☐ ☐ ☐
☐ ☐ ☐

GRATITUDE

NOTES

_____
_____
_____
_____
_____
_____
_____
_____
_____
_____

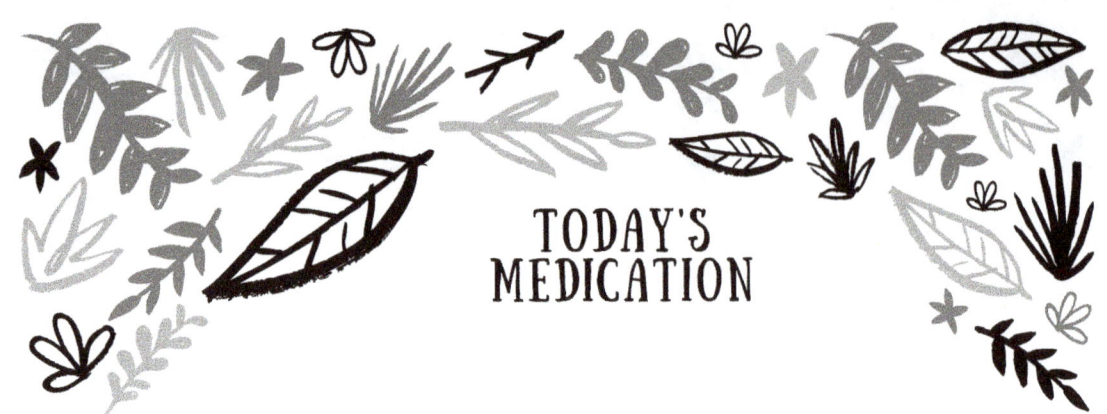

TODAY'S MEDICATION

TIME	MEDICATION	DOSAGE	REACTIONS

DATE _____
CHEMO DRUG _____
DAY # _____ AFTER CHEMO # _____

TODAY I FEEL

_____
_____
_____

EXERCISE
☐
☐
☐

FOOD & DRINK
☐
☐
☐

SLEEP
☐
☐
☐

GRATITUDE

○ ○ ○ ○ ○ ○

NOTES
_____
_____
_____
_____
_____
_____
_____
_____
_____
_____

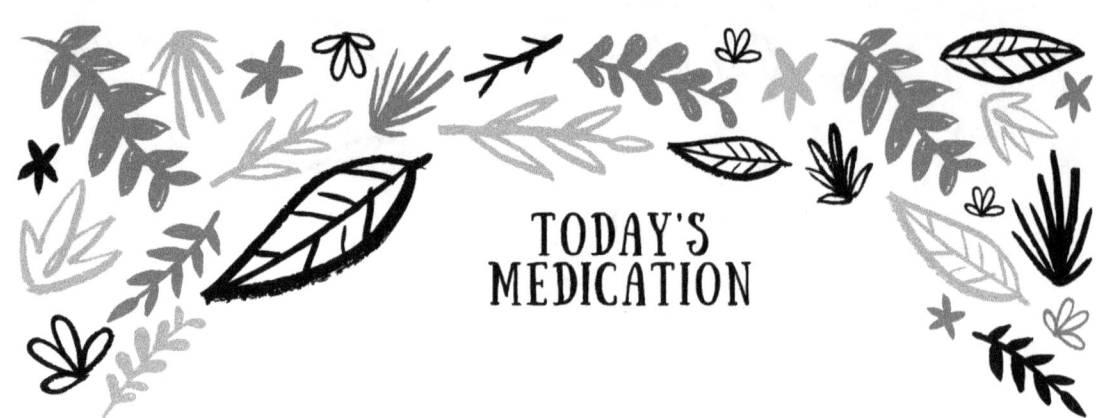

TODAY'S MEDICATION

TIME	MEDICATION	DOSAGE	REACTIONS

DATE _____
CHEMO DRUG _____
DAY# _____ AFTER CHEMO # _____

TODAY I FEEL

_____
_____
_____

EXERCISE   **FOOD & DRINK**   **SLEEP**
☐ ☐ ☐
☐ ☐ ☐
☐ ☐ ☐

GRATITUDE   **NOTES**
_____
_____
_____
_____
_____
_____
_____
_____
_____
_____

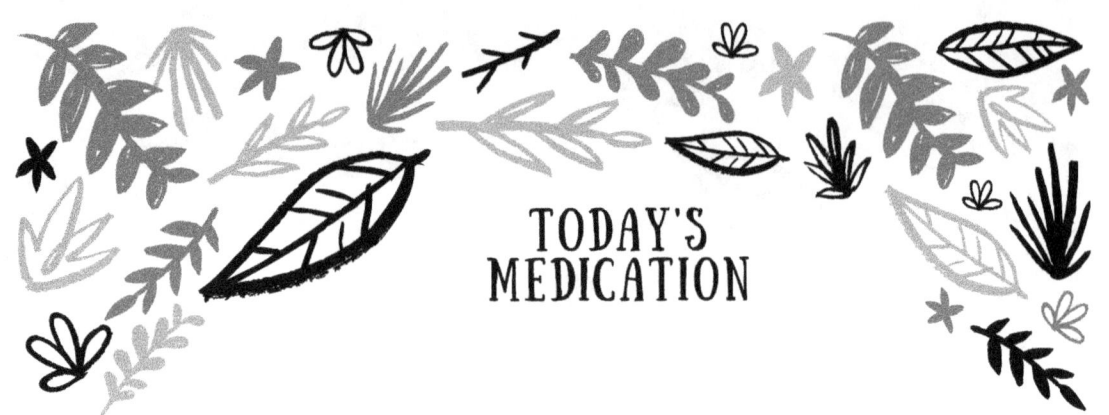

TODAY'S MEDICATION

TIME	MEDICATION	DOSAGE	REACTIONS

DATE _____
CHEMO DRUG _____
DAY# _____ AFTER CHEMO # _____

TODAY I FEEL

_____
_____
_____
_____

EXERCISE   **FOOD & DRINK**   **SLEEP**
☐ ☐ ☐
☐ ☐ ☐
☐ ☐ ☐

GRATITUDE   **NOTES**
_____
_____
_____
_____
_____
_____
_____
_____
_____
_____

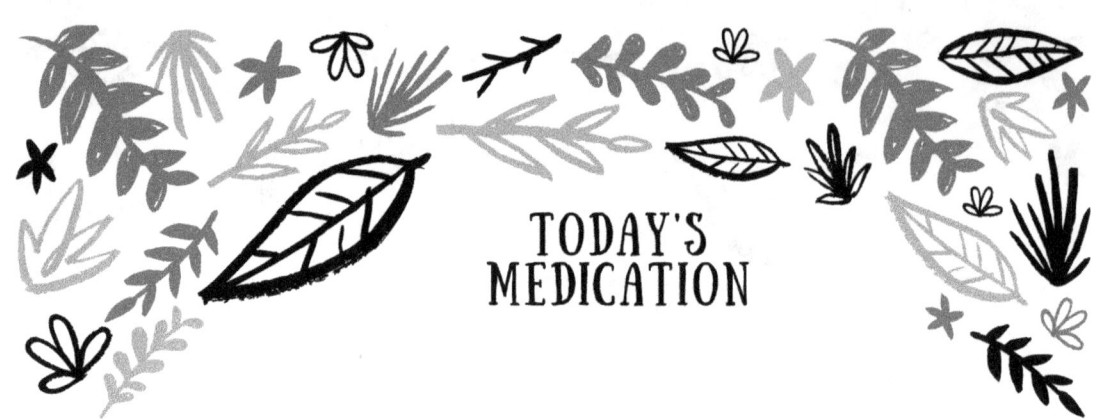

TODAY'S MEDICATION

TIME	MEDICATION	DOSAGE	REACTIONS

DATE _____

CHEMO DRUG _____

DAY # _____ AFTER CHEMO # _____

TODAY I FEEL

_____
_____
_____
_____

EXERCISE
- [ ]
- [ ]
- [ ]

FOOD & DRINK
- [ ]
- [ ]
- [ ]

SLEEP
- [ ]
- [ ]
- [ ]

◯ ◯ ◯ ◯ ◯ ◯

GRATITUDE

NOTES

_____
_____
_____
_____
_____
_____
_____
_____
_____
_____
_____

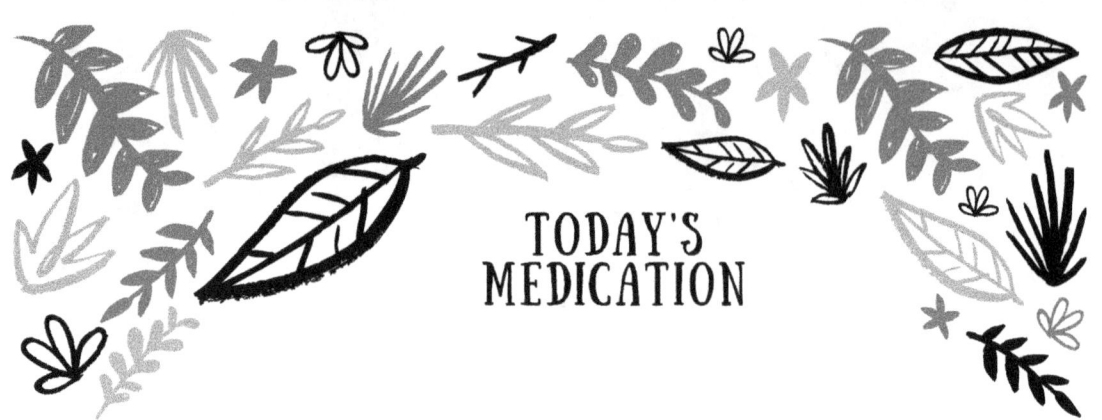

TODAY'S MEDICATION

TIME	MEDICATION	DOSAGE	REACTIONS

DATE _____

CHEMO DRUG _____

DAY # _____ AFTER CHEMO # _____

TODAY I FEEL

_____
_____
_____
_____

EXERCISE
☐
☐
☐

FOOD & DRINK
☐
☐
☐

SLEEP
☐
☐
☐

GRATITUDE

NOTES

_____
_____
_____
_____
_____
_____
_____
_____
_____
_____

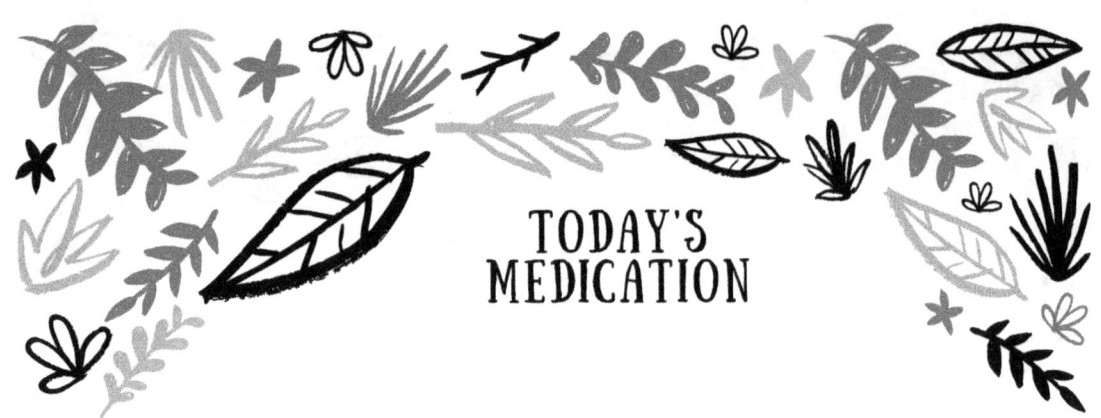

TODAY'S MEDICATION

TIME	MEDICATION	DOSAGE	REACTIONS

DATE _____
CHEMO DRUG _____
DAY# _____ AFTER CHEMO # _____

TODAY I FEEL

_____
_____
_____
_____

EXERCISE
☐
☐
☐

FOOD & DRINK
☐
☐
☐

SLEEP
☐
☐
☐

GRATITUDE

NOTES

_____
_____
_____
_____
_____
_____
_____
_____
_____
_____
_____

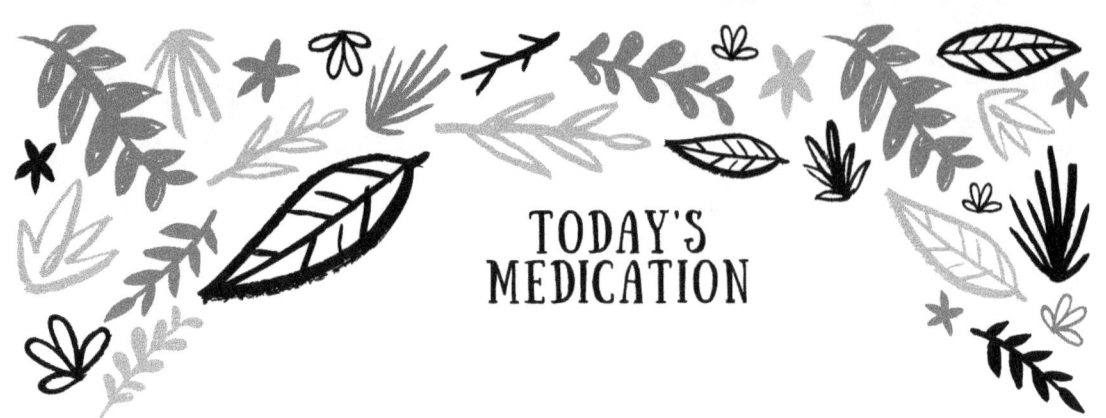

TODAY'S MEDICATION

TIME	MEDICATION	DOSAGE	REACTIONS

DATE _____
CHEMO DRUG _____
DAY # _____ AFTER CHEMO # _____

TODAY I FEEL

_____
_____
_____
_____

EXERCISE
☐
☐
☐

FOOD & DRINK
☐
☐
☐

SLEEP
☐
☐
☐

GRATITUDE

NOTES
_____
_____
_____
_____
_____
_____
_____
_____
_____
_____
_____

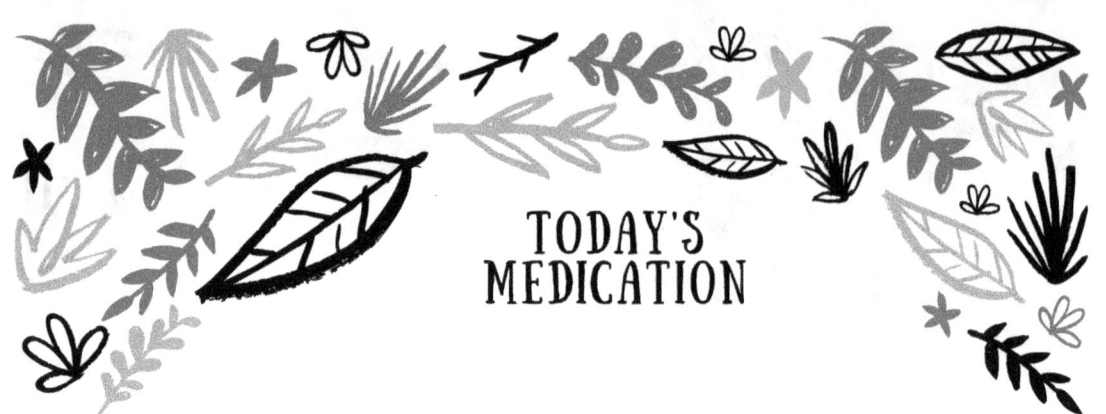

TIME	MEDICATION	DOSAGE	REACTIONS

DATE _____
CHEMO DRUG _____
DAY# _____ AFTER CHEMO # _____

TODAY I FEEL

_____
_____
_____
_____

EXERCISE **FOOD & DRINK** **SLEEP**
☐ ☐ ☐
☐ ☐ ☐
☐ ☐ ☐

GRATITUDE **NOTES**

_____
_____
_____
_____
_____
_____
_____
_____
_____
_____

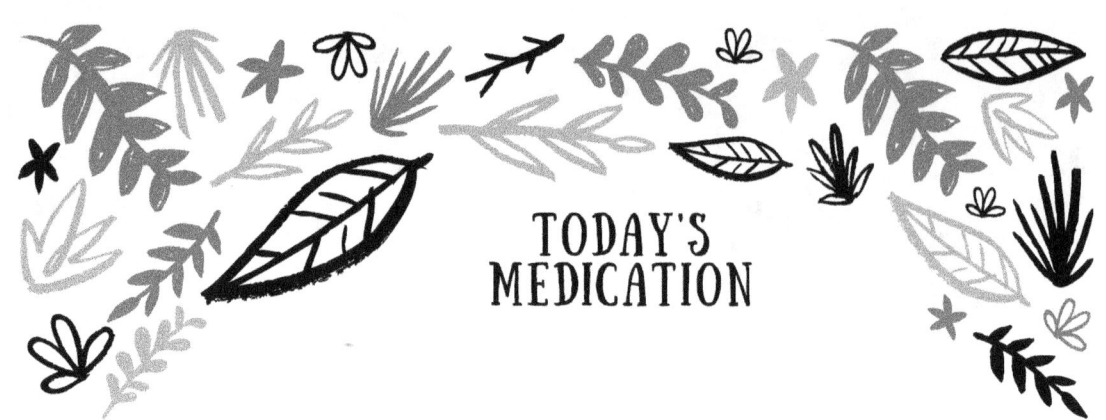

TODAY'S MEDICATION

TIME	MEDICATION	DOSAGE	REACTIONS

DATE _____

CHEMO DRUG _____

DAY # _____ AFTER CHEMO # _____

TODAY I FEEL

_____
_____
_____
_____

EXERCISE
☐
☐
☐

FOOD & DRINK
☐
☐
☐

SLEEP
☐
☐
☐

GRATITUDE

NOTES
_____
_____
_____
_____
_____
_____
_____
_____
_____
_____

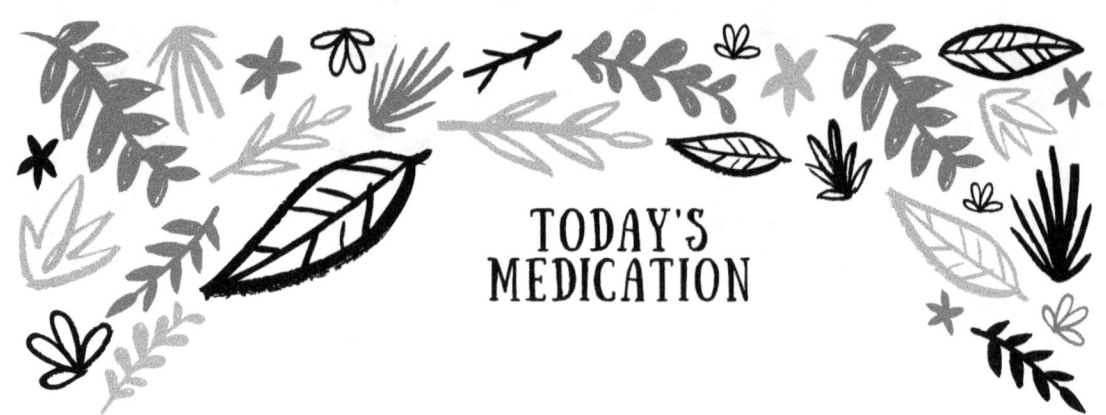

TODAY'S MEDICATION

TIME	MEDICATION	DOSAGE	REACTIONS

DATE _____
CHEMO DRUG _____
DAY # _____ AFTER CHEMO # _____

TODAY I FEEL

_____
_____
_____
_____

EXERCISE **FOOD & DRINK** **SLEEP**
☐ ☐ ☐
☐ ☐ ☐
☐ ☐ ☐

GRATITUDE **NOTES**
_____
_____
_____
_____
_____
_____
_____
_____
_____
_____

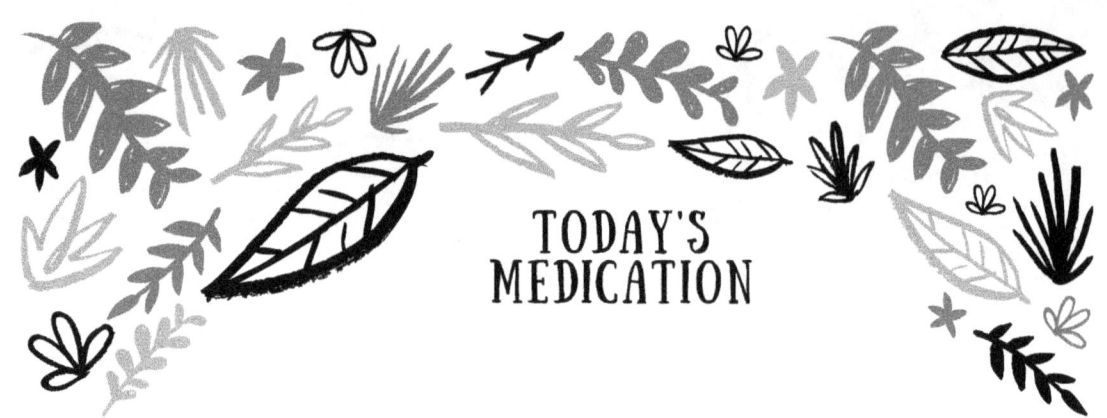

TODAY'S MEDICATION

TIME	MEDICATION	DOSAGE	REACTIONS

DATE _____
CHEMO DRUG _____
DAY # _____ AFTER CHEMO # _____

TODAY I FEEL

_____
_____
_____
_____

EXERCISE
☐
☐
☐

FOOD & DRINK
☐
☐
☐

SLEEP
☐
☐
☐

GRATITUDE

NOTES
_____
_____
_____
_____
_____
_____
_____
_____
_____
_____

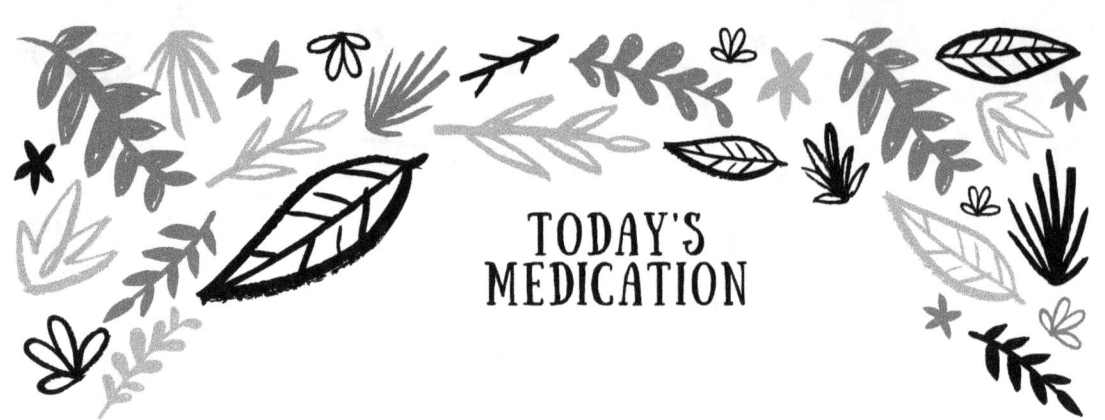

TODAY'S MEDICATION

TIME	MEDICATION	DOSAGE	REACTIONS

DATE _____

CHEMO DRUG _____

DAY # _____ AFTER CHEMO # _____

TODAY I FEEL

_____
_____
_____
_____

EXERCISE
☐
☐
☐

FOOD & DRINK
☐
☐
☐

SLEEP
☐
☐
☐

GRATITUDE

◯ ◯ ◯ ◯ ◯ ◯

NOTES

_____
_____
_____
_____
_____
_____
_____
_____
_____
_____

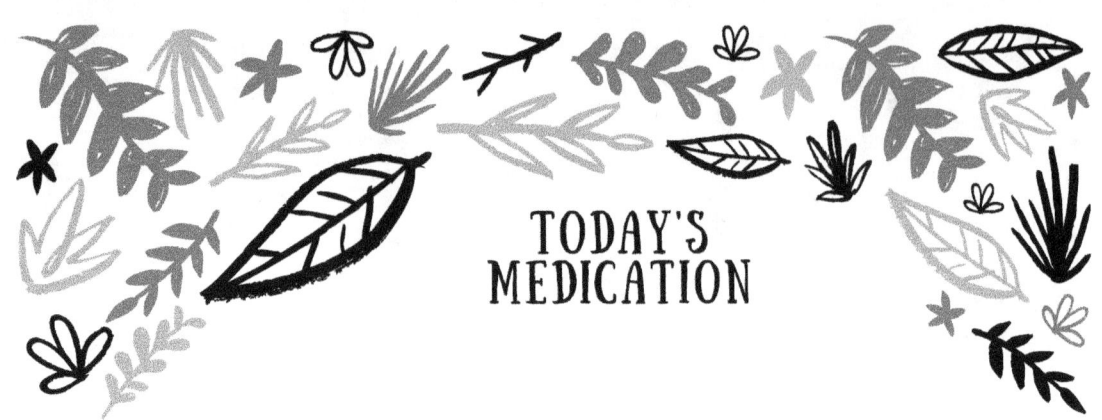

TODAY'S MEDICATION

TIME	MEDICATION	DOSAGE	REACTIONS

DATE _____
CHEMO DRUG _____
DAY # _____ AFTER CHEMO # _____

TODAY I FEEL

_____
_____
_____
_____

EXERCISE
☐
☐
☐

FOOD & DRINK
☐
☐
☐

SLEEP
☐
☐
☐

GRATITUDE

NOTES
_____
_____
_____
_____
_____
_____
_____
_____
_____
_____

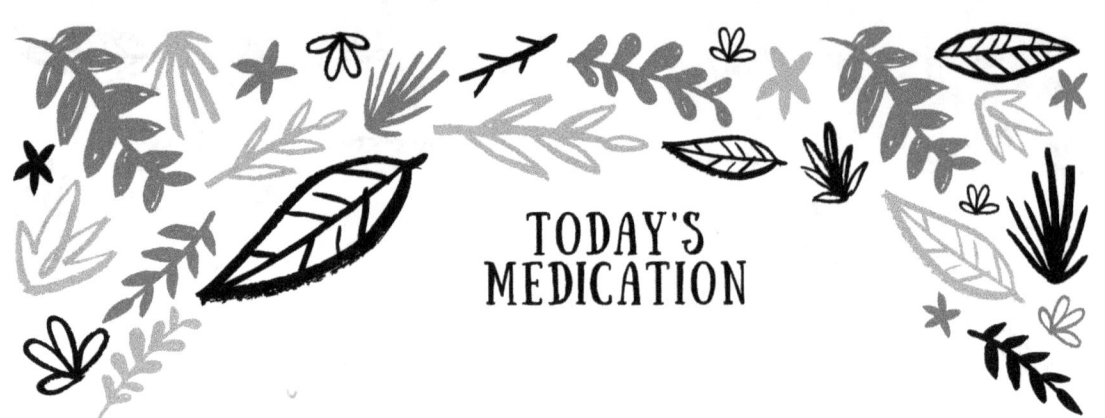

TODAY'S MEDICATION

TIME	MEDICATION	DOSAGE	REACTIONS

DATE _____

CHEMO DRUG _____

DAY # _____ AFTER CHEMO # _____

TODAY I FEEL

_____
_____
_____

EXERCISE
☐
☐
☐

FOOD & DRINK
☐
☐
☐

SLEEP
☐
☐
☐

GRATITUDE

NOTES
_____
_____
_____
_____
_____
_____
_____
_____
_____
_____

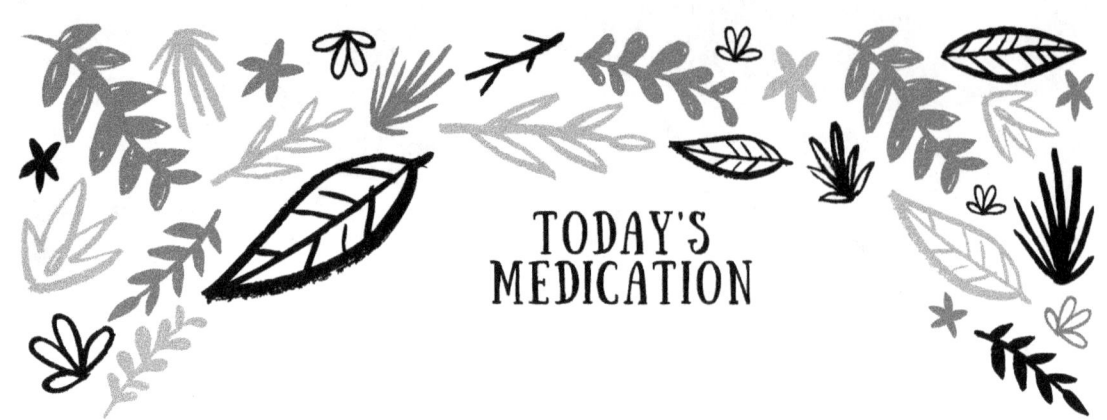

TODAY'S MEDICATION

TIME	MEDICATION	DOSAGE	REACTIONS

DATE _____
CHEMO DRUG _____
DAY # _____ AFTER CHEMO # _____

TODAY I FEEL

_____
_____
_____
_____

EXERCISE   **FOOD & DRINK**   **SLEEP**
☐   ☐   ☐
☐   ☐   ☐
☐   ☐   ☐

◯ ◯ ◯ ◯ ◯ ◯

GRATITUDE   **NOTES**
_____
_____
_____
_____
_____
_____
_____
_____
_____

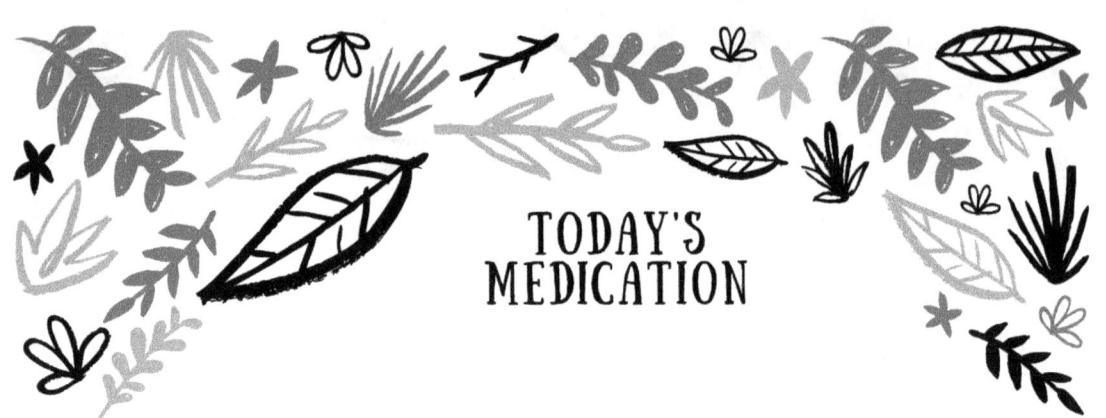

TODAY'S MEDICATION

TIME	MEDICATION	DOSAGE	REACTIONS

DATE _____
CHEMO DRUG _____
DAY # _____ AFTER CHEMO # _____

TODAY I FEEL

_____
_____
_____
_____

EXERCISE
☐
☐
☐

FOOD & DRINK
☐
☐
☐

SLEEP
☐
☐
☐

GRATITUDE

NOTES
_____
_____
_____
_____
_____
_____
_____
_____
_____
_____
_____

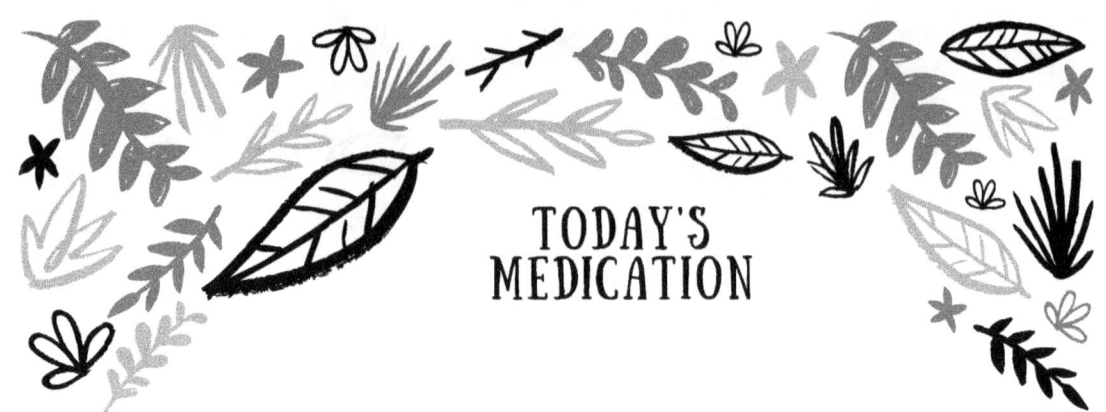

TODAY'S MEDICATION

TIME	MEDICATION	DOSAGE	REACTIONS

DATE _____
CHEMO DRUG _____
DAY# _____ AFTER CHEMO # _____

TODAY I FEEL

_____
_____
_____
_____

EXERCISE **FOOD & DRINK** **SLEEP**
☐   ☐   ☐
☐   ☐   ☐
☐   ☐   ☐

GRATITUDE   ◯ ◯ ◯ ◯ ◯ ◯

NOTES
_____
_____
_____
_____
_____
_____
_____
_____
_____
_____

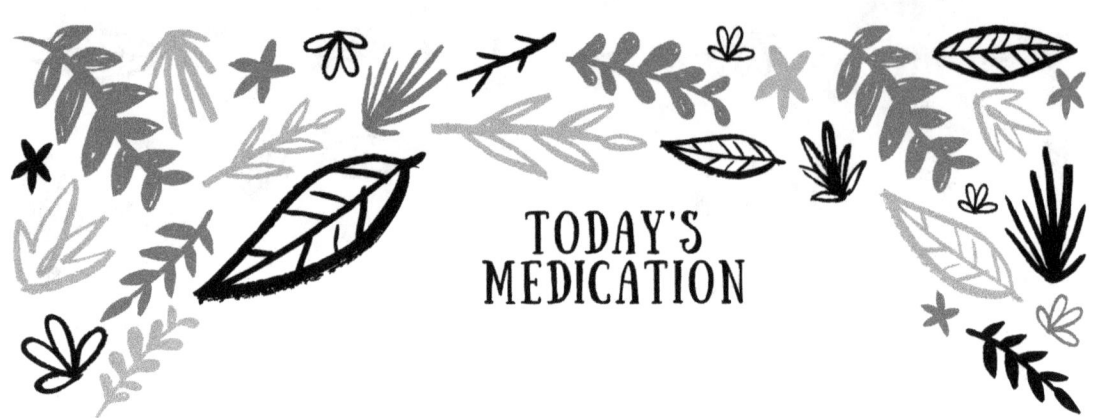

TODAY'S MEDICATION

TIME	MEDICATION	DOSAGE	REACTIONS

DATE _____
CHEMO DRUG _____
DAY # _____ AFTER CHEMO # _____

TODAY I FEEL

_____
_____
_____
_____

EXERCISE
☐
☐
☐

FOOD & DRINK
☐
☐
☐

SLEEP
☐
☐
☐

GRATITUDE

NOTES
_____
_____
_____
_____
_____
_____
_____
_____
_____
_____
_____

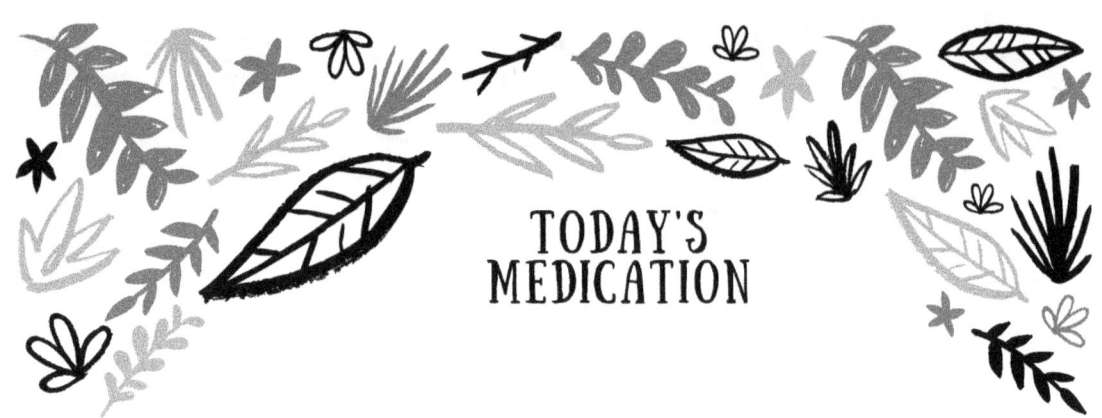

TODAY'S MEDICATION

TIME	MEDICATION	DOSAGE	REACTIONS

DATE _____
CHEMO DRUG _____
DAY# _____ AFTER CHEMO # _____

TODAY I FEEL

_____
_____
_____

EXERCISE **FOOD & DRINK** **SLEEP**
☐ ☐ ☐
☐ ☐ ☐
☐ ☐ ☐

GRATITUDE **NOTES**
_____
_____
_____
_____
_____
_____
_____
_____
_____

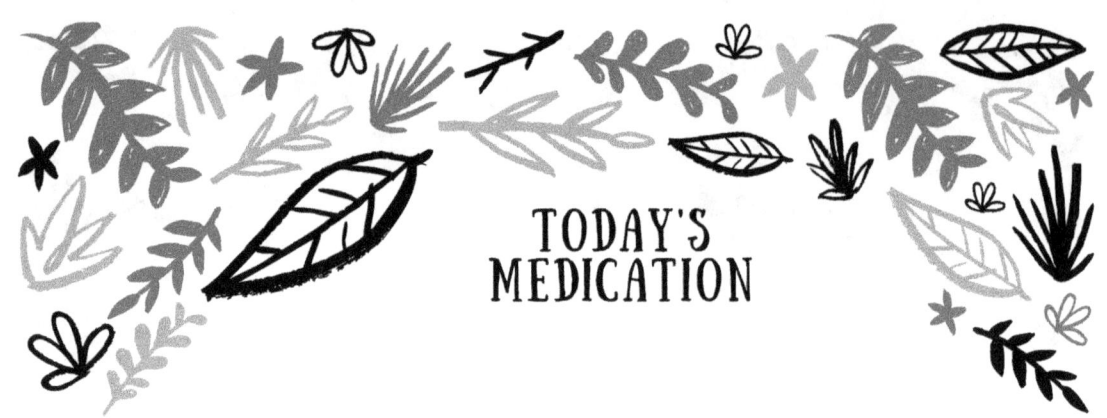

TODAY'S MEDICATION

TIME	MEDICATION	DOSAGE	REACTIONS

DATE _____
CHEMO DRUG _____
DAY # _____ AFTER CHEMO # _____

TODAY I FEEL

_____
_____
_____
_____

EXERCISE
☐
☐
☐

FOOD & DRINK
☐
☐
☐

SLEEP
☐
☐
☐

GRATITUDE

NOTES
_____
_____
_____
_____
_____
_____
_____
_____
_____
_____

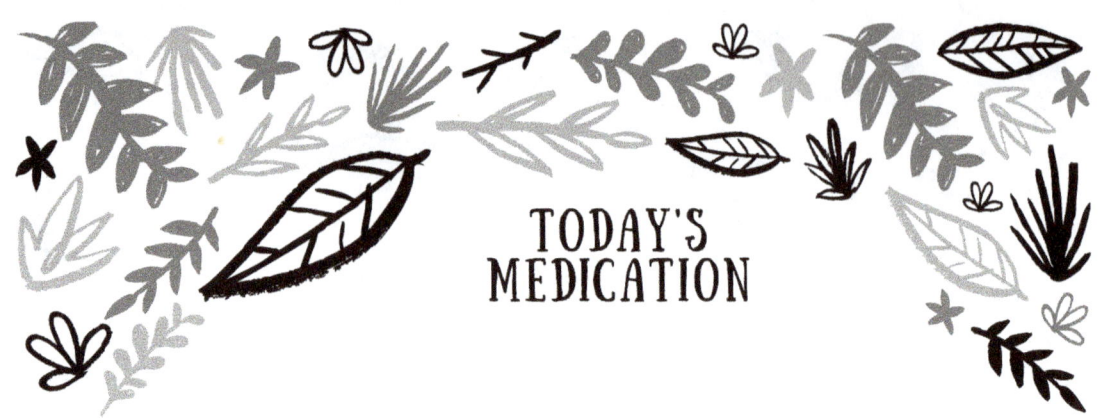

TODAY'S MEDICATION

TIME	MEDICATION	DOSAGE	REACTIONS

DATE _____
CHEMO DRUG _____
DAY# _____ AFTER CHEMO # _____

TODAY I FEEL

_____
_____
_____
_____

EXERCISE
☐
☐
☐

FOOD & DRINK
☐
☐
☐

SLEEP
☐
☐
☐

GRATITUDE

NOTES
_____
_____
_____
_____
_____
_____
_____
_____
_____
_____

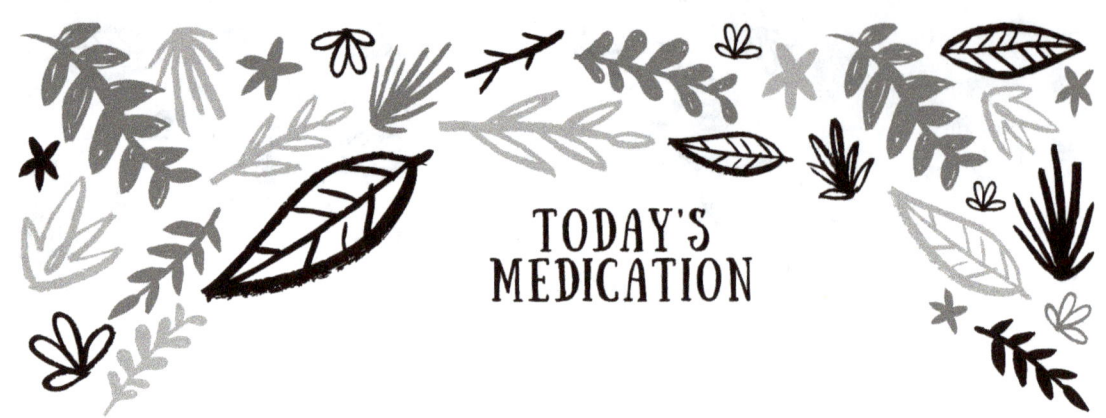

TODAY'S MEDICATION

TIME	MEDICATION	DOSAGE	REACTIONS

DATE _____
CHEMO DRUG _____
DAY # _____ AFTER CHEMO # _____

TODAY I FEEL

_____
_____
_____
_____

EXERCISE
☐
☐
☐

FOOD & DRINK
☐
☐
☐

SLEEP
☐
☐
☐

GRATITUDE

NOTES
_____
_____
_____
_____
_____
_____
_____
_____
_____
_____
_____

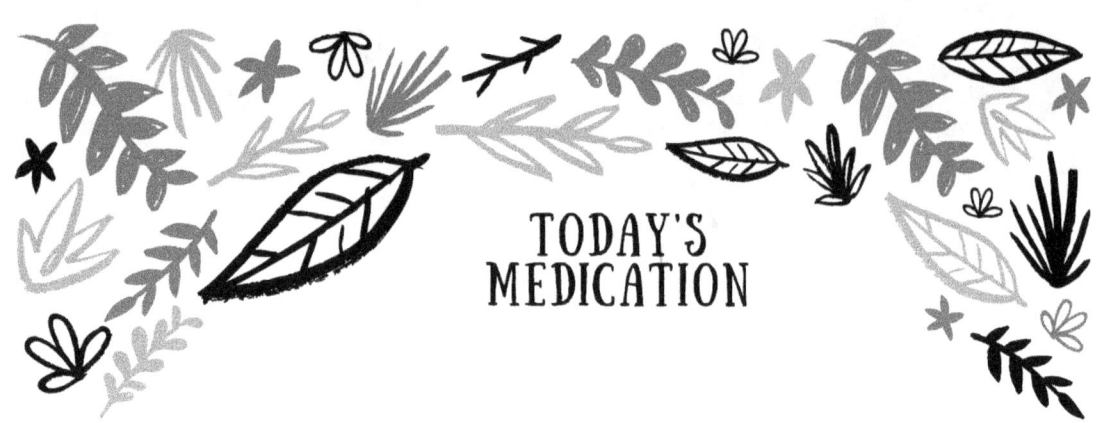

TODAY'S MEDICATION

TIME	MEDICATION	DOSAGE	REACTIONS

DATE _____
CHEMO DRUG _____
DAY# _____ AFTER CHEMO # _____

TODAY I FEEL

_____
_____
_____
_____

EXERCISE **FOOD & DRINK** **SLEEP**
☐ ☐ ☐
☐ ☐ ☐
☐ ☐ ☐

GRATITUDE **NOTES**

_____
_____
_____
_____
_____
_____
_____
_____
_____
_____

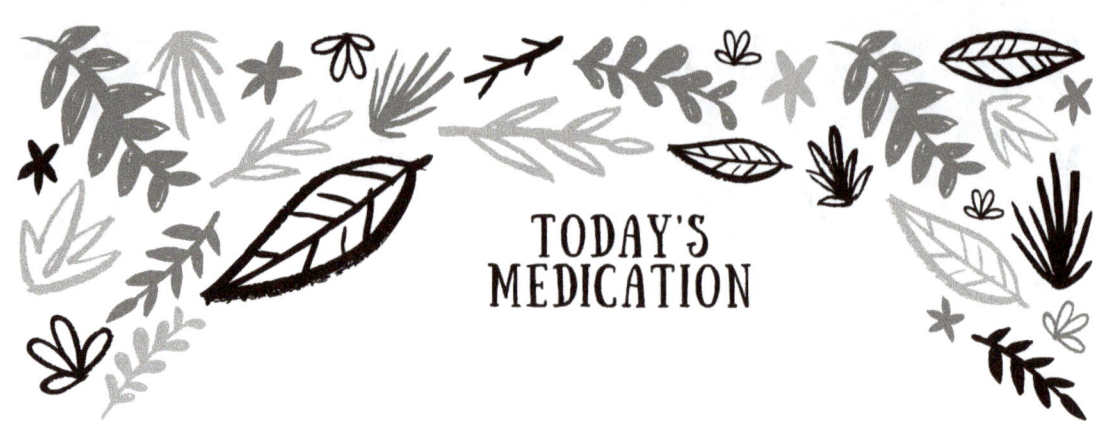

TODAY'S MEDICATION

TIME	MEDICATION	DOSAGE	REACTIONS

DATE _____
CHEMO DRUG _____
DAY # _____ AFTER CHEMO # _____

TODAY I FEEL

_____
_____
_____
_____

EXERCISE **FOOD & DRINK** **SLEEP**
☐ ☐ ☐
☐ ☐ ☐
☐ ☐ ☐

GRATITUDE

◯ ◯ ◯ ◯ ◯ ◯

NOTES

_____
_____
_____
_____
_____
_____
_____
_____
_____
_____

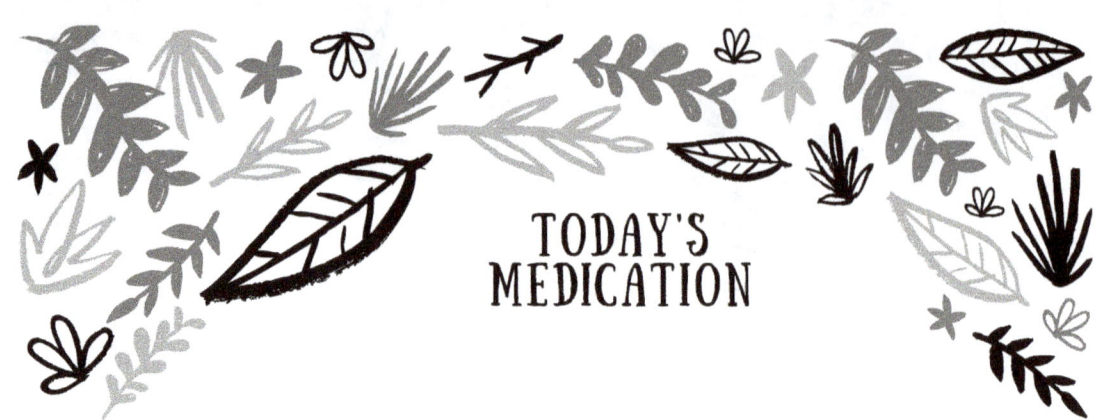

TODAY'S MEDICATION

TIME	MEDICATION	DOSAGE	REACTIONS

DATE _____
CHEMO DRUG _____
DAY # _____ AFTER CHEMO # _____

TODAY I FEEL

_____
_____
_____
_____

EXERCISE
☐
☐
☐

FOOD & DRINK
☐
☐
☐

SLEEP
☐
☐
☐

GRATITUDE

◯ ◯ ◯ ◯ ◯ ◯

NOTES
_____
_____
_____
_____
_____
_____
_____
_____
_____
_____

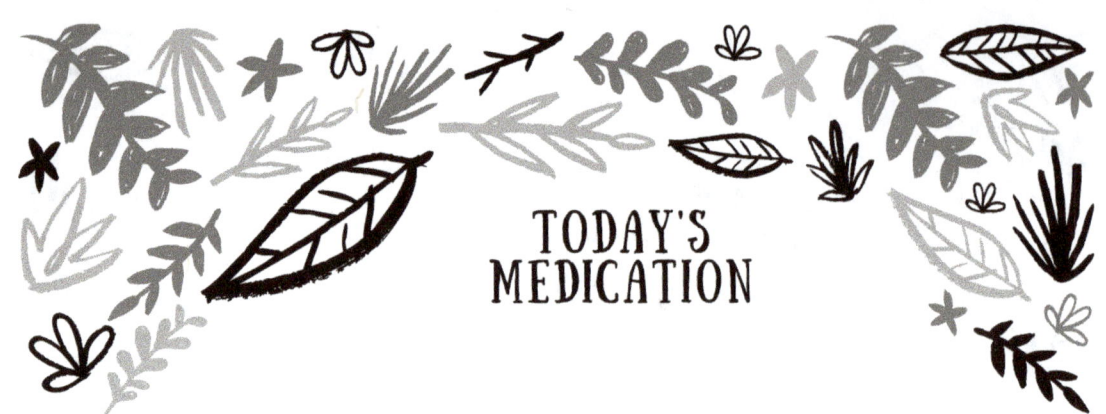

TODAY'S MEDICATION

TIME	MEDICATION	DOSAGE	REACTIONS

DATE _____
CHEMO DRUG _____
DAY # _____ AFTER CHEMO # _____

TODAY I FEEL

_____
_____
_____
_____

EXERCISE
☐
☐
☐

FOOD & DRINK
☐
☐
☐

SLEEP
☐
☐
☐

GRATITUDE

NOTES
_____
_____
_____
_____
_____
_____
_____
_____
_____
_____
_____

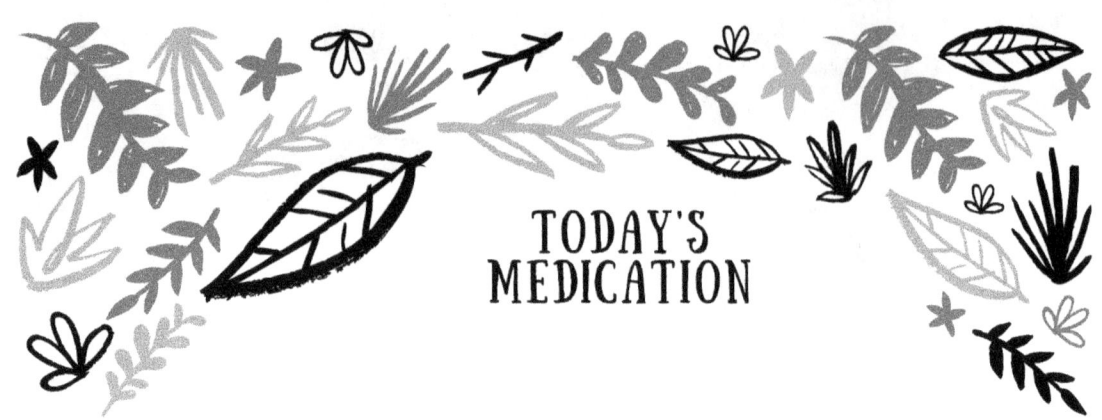

TODAY'S MEDICATION

TIME	MEDICATION	DOSAGE	REACTIONS

DATE _____
CHEMO DRUG _____
DAY # _____ AFTER CHEMO # _____

TODAY I FEEL

_____
_____
_____
_____

EXERCISE
☐
☐
☐

FOOD & DRINK
☐
☐
☐

SLEEP
☐
☐
☐

GRATITUDE

NOTES
_____
_____
_____
_____
_____
_____
_____
_____
_____
_____
_____

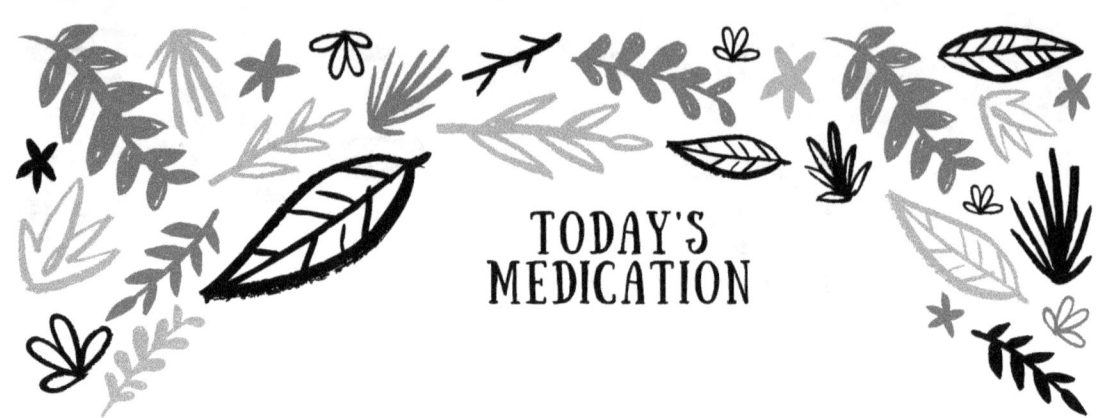

TODAY'S MEDICATION

TIME	MEDICATION	DOSAGE	REACTIONS

DATE _____
CHEMO DRUG _____
DAY # _____ AFTER CHEMO # _____

TODAY I FEEL

_____
_____
_____
_____

EXERCISE **FOOD & DRINK** **SLEEP**
☐ ☐ ☐
☐ ☐ ☐
☐ ☐ ☐

GRATITUDE

NOTES

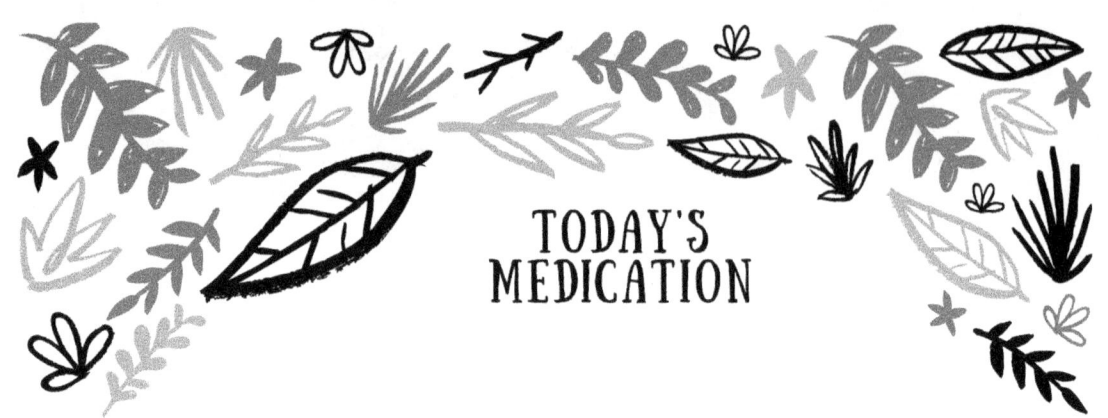

TODAY'S MEDICATION

TIME	MEDICATION	DOSAGE	REACTIONS

DATE _____
CHEMO DRUG _____
DAY # _____ AFTER CHEMO # _____

TODAY I FEEL

_____
_____
_____

EXERCISE
☐
☐
☐

FOOD & DRINK
☐
☐
☐

SLEEP
☐
☐
☐

GRATITUDE

NOTES
_____
_____
_____
_____
_____
_____
_____
_____
_____

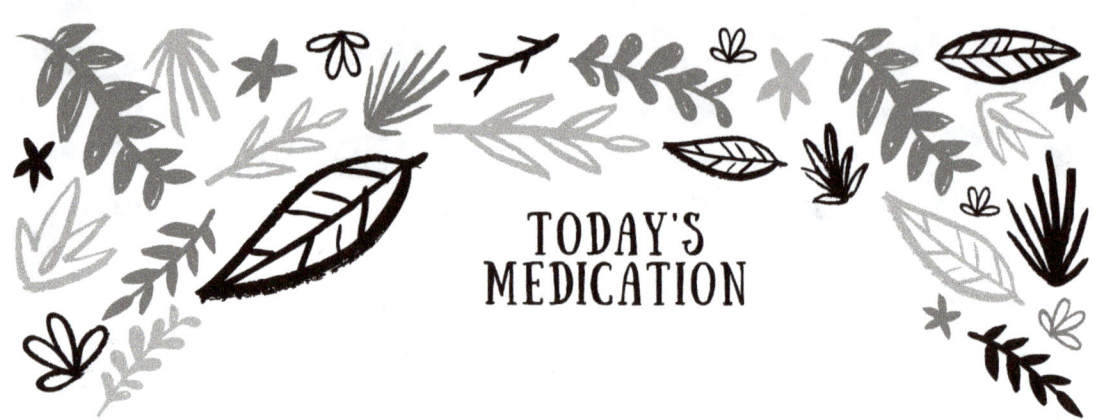

TODAY'S MEDICATION

TIME	MEDICATION	DOSAGE	REACTIONS

DATE _____
CHEMO DRUG _____
DAY # _____ AFTER CHEMO # _____

TODAY I FEEL

_____
_____
_____
_____

EXERCISE
☐
☐
☐

FOOD & DRINK
☐
☐
☐

SLEEP
☐
☐
☐

GRATITUDE

⬤ ⬤ ⬤ ⬤ ⬤ ⬤

NOTES
_____
_____
_____
_____
_____
_____
_____
_____
_____
_____
_____

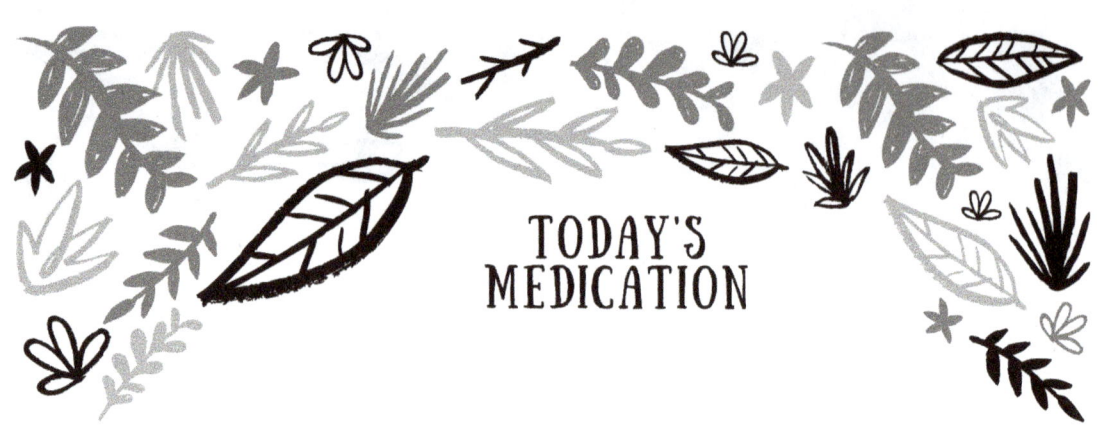

TODAY'S MEDICATION

TIME	MEDICATION	DOSAGE	REACTIONS

DATE _____
CHEMO DRUG _____
DAY# _____ AFTER CHEMO # _____

TODAY I FEEL

_____
_____
_____
_____

EXERCISE **FOOD & DRINK** **SLEEP**
☐ ☐ ☐
☐ ☐ ☐
☐ ☐ ☐

GRATITUDE **NOTES**
_____
_____
_____
_____
_____
_____
_____
_____
_____
_____

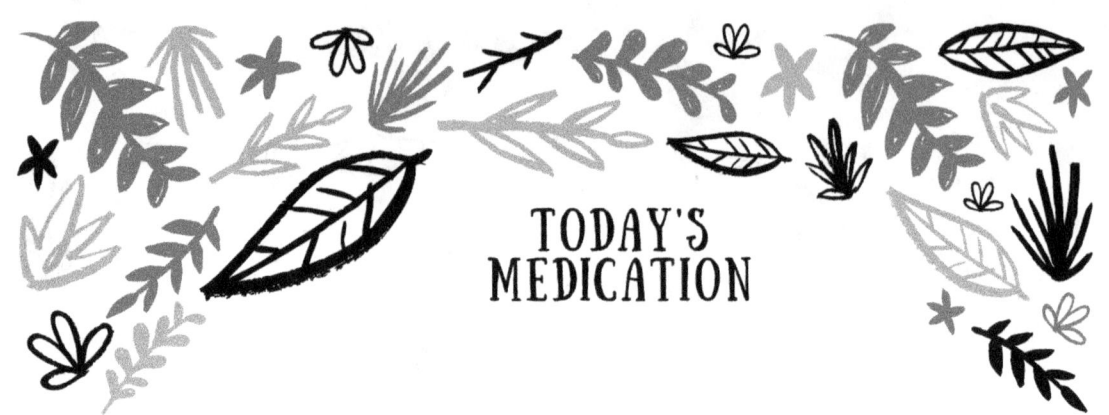

TODAY'S MEDICATION

TIME	MEDICATION	DOSAGE	REACTIONS

DATE _____

CHEMO DRUG _____

DAY# _____ AFTER CHEMO # _____

TODAY I FEEL

_____
_____
_____
_____

EXERCISE
☐
☐
☐

FOOD & DRINK
☐
☐
☐

SLEEP
☐
☐
☐

GRATITUDE

NOTES
_____
_____
_____
_____
_____
_____
_____
_____
_____
_____
_____

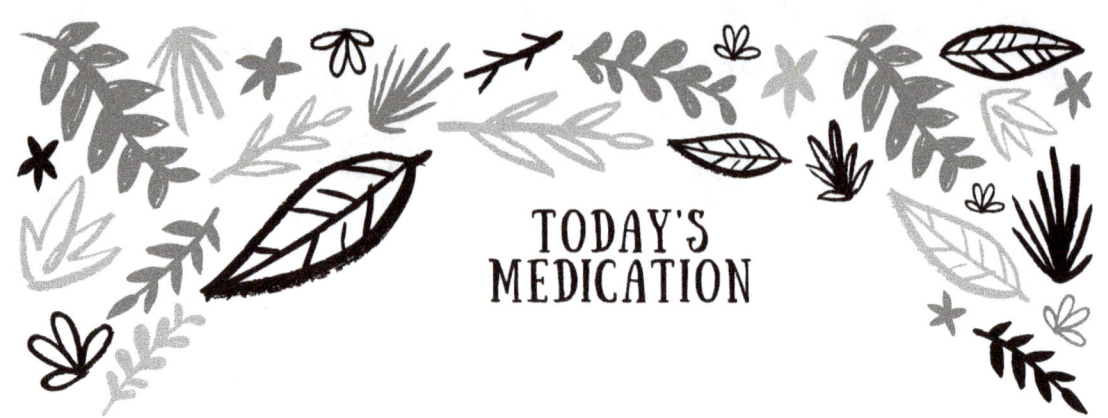

TODAY'S MEDICATION

TIME	MEDICATION	DOSAGE	REACTIONS

DATE _____
CHEMO DRUG _____
DAY # _____ AFTER CHEMO # _____

TODAY I FEEL

_____
_____
_____
_____

EXERCISE
☐
☐
☐

FOOD & DRINK
☐
☐
☐

SLEEP
☐
☐
☐

GRATITUDE

NOTES
_____
_____
_____
_____
_____
_____
_____
_____
_____
_____

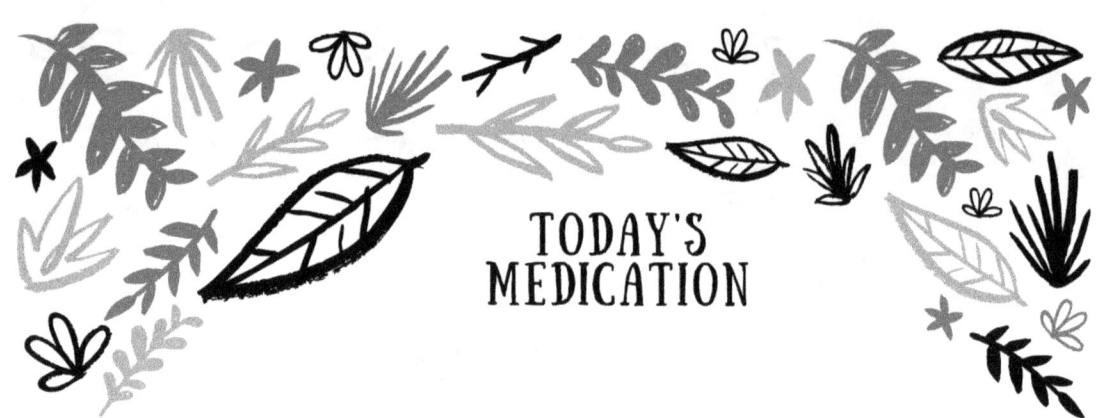

TODAY'S MEDICATION

TIME	MEDICATION	DOSAGE	REACTIONS

DATE _____
CHEMO DRUG _____
DAY # _____ AFTER CHEMO # _____

TODAY I FEEL

_____
_____
_____
_____

EXERCISE
☐
☐
☐

FOOD & DRINK
☐
☐
☐

SLEEP
☐
☐
☐

GRATITUDE

NOTES
_____
_____
_____
_____
_____
_____
_____
_____
_____
_____
_____
_____

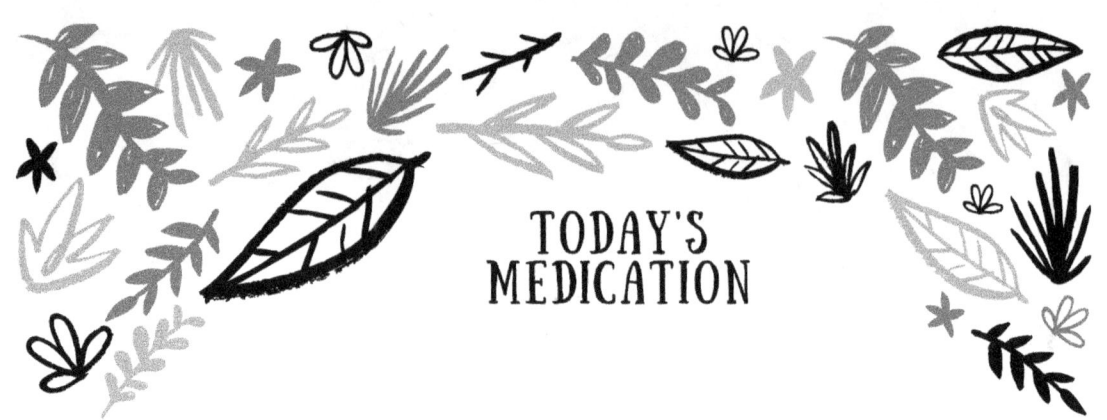

TODAY'S MEDICATION

TIME	MEDICATION	DOSAGE	REACTIONS

DATE _____
CHEMO DRUG _____
DAY # _____ AFTER CHEMO # _____

TODAY I FEEL

_____
_____
_____

EXERCISE
☐
☐
☐

FOOD & DRINK
☐
☐
☐

SLEEP
☐
☐
☐

GRATITUDE

NOTES
_____
_____
_____
_____
_____
_____
_____
_____
_____

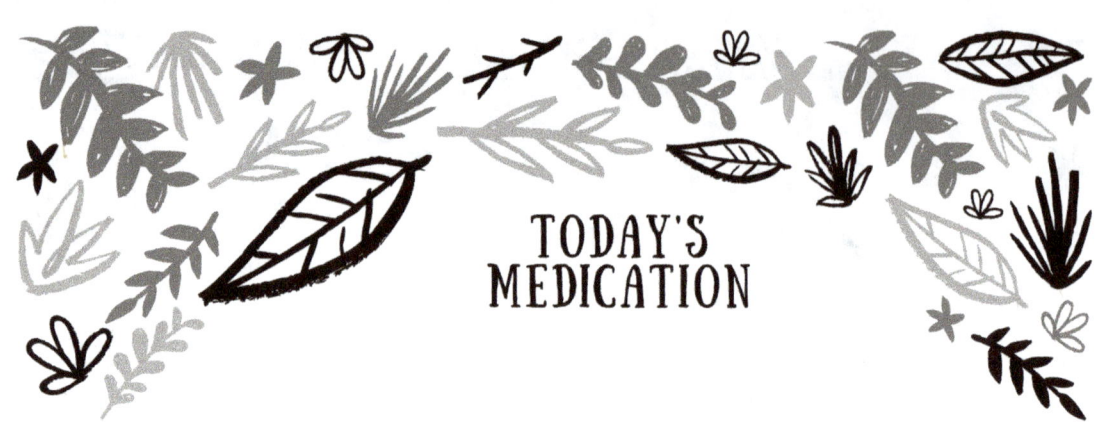

Today's Medication

TIME	MEDICATION	DOSAGE	REACTIONS

DATE _____
CHEMO DRUG _____
DAY # _____ AFTER CHEMO # _____

TODAY I FEEL

_____
_____
_____
_____

EXERCISE **FOOD & DRINK** **SLEEP**

☐ ☐ ☐
☐ ☐ ☐
☐ ☐ ☐

GRATITUDE

NOTES

_____
_____
_____
_____
_____
_____
_____
_____
_____
_____
_____

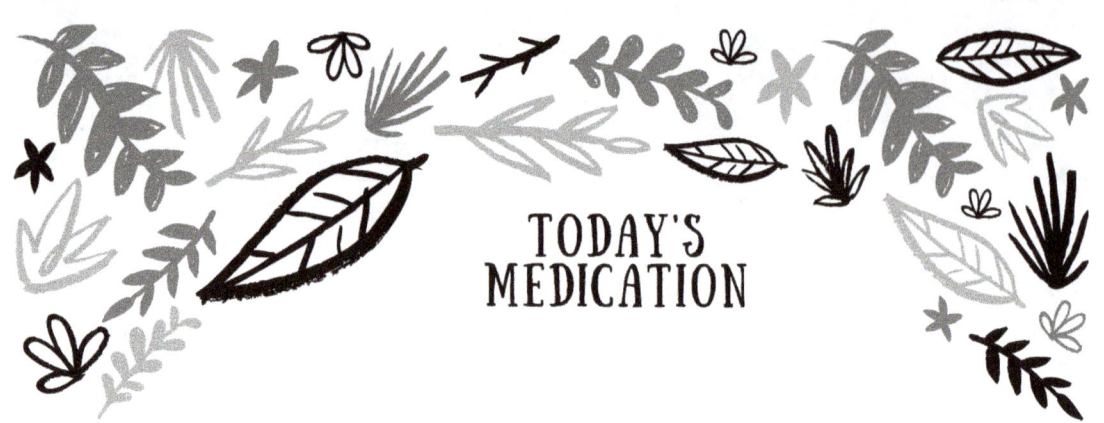

TODAY'S MEDICATION

TIME	MEDICATION	DOSAGE	REACTIONS

DATE _____
CHEMO DRUG _____
DAY # _____ AFTER CHEMO # _____

TODAY I FEEL

_____
_____
_____

EXERCISE
☐
☐
☐

FOOD & DRINK
☐
☐
☐

SLEEP
☐
☐
☐

GRATITUDE

NOTES
_____
_____
_____
_____
_____
_____
_____
_____
_____
_____

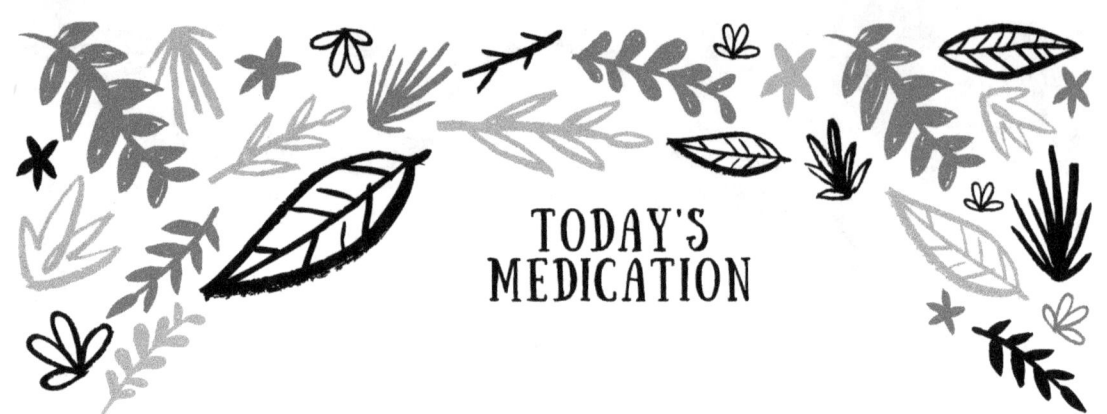

TODAY'S MEDICATION

TIME	MEDICATION	DOSAGE	REACTIONS

DATE _____
CHEMO DRUG _____
DAY # _____ AFTER CHEMO # _____

TODAY I FEEL

_____
_____
_____
_____

EXERCISE **FOOD & DRINK** **SLEEP**
☐ ☐ ☐
☐ ☐ ☐
☐ ☐ ☐

GRATITUDE

○ ○ ○ ○ ○ ○

NOTES

_____
_____
_____
_____
_____
_____
_____
_____
_____
_____
_____

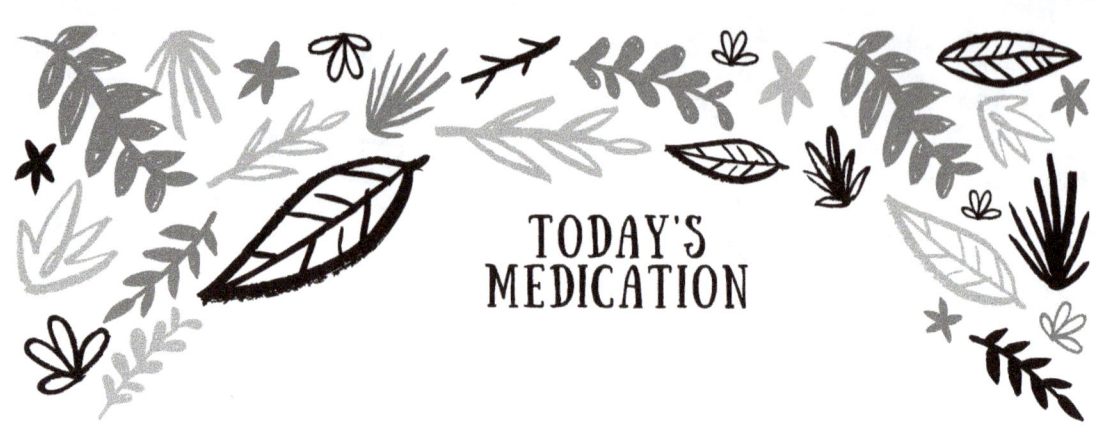

TODAY'S MEDICATION

TIME	MEDICATION	DOSAGE	REACTIONS

DATE _____
CHEMO DRUG _____
DAY # _____ AFTER CHEMO # _____

TODAY I FEEL

_____
_____
_____
_____

EXERCISE
☐
☐
☐

FOOD & DRINK
☐
☐
☐

SLEEP
☐
☐
☐

GRATITUDE

NOTES
_____
_____
_____
_____
_____
_____
_____
_____
_____
_____
_____

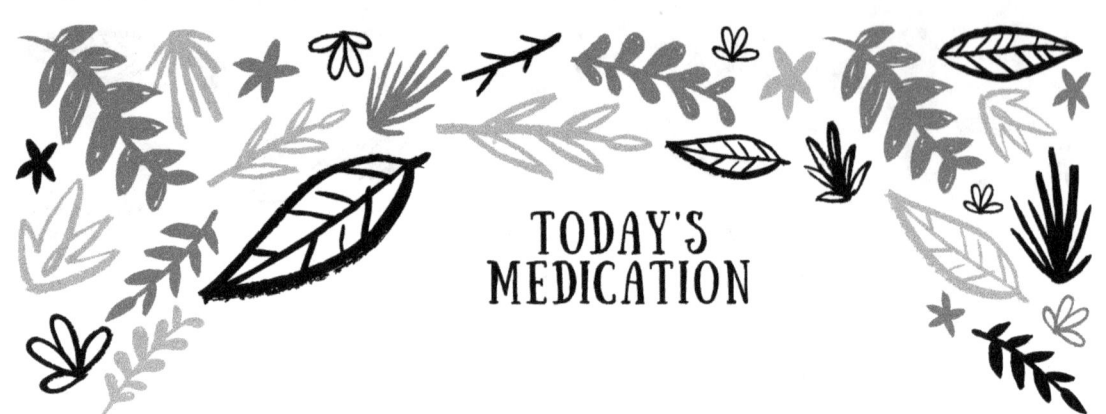

TODAY'S MEDICATION

TIME	MEDICATION	DOSAGE	REACTIONS

DATE _____
CHEMO DRUG _____
DAY # _____ AFTER CHEMO # _____

TODAY I FEEL

_____
_____
_____
_____

EXERCISE
☐
☐
☐

FOOD & DRINK
☐
☐
☐

SLEEP
☐
☐
☐

GRATITUDE

○ ○ ○ ○ ○ ○

NOTES
_____
_____
_____
_____
_____
_____
_____
_____
_____
_____

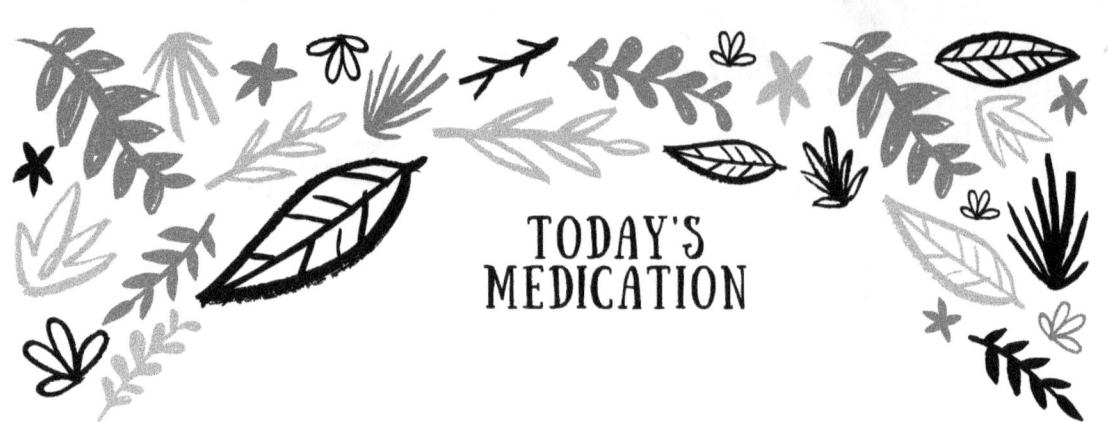

TODAY'S MEDICATION

TIME	MEDICATION	DOSAGE	REACTIONS

www.ingramcontent.com/pod-product-compliance
Lightning Source LLC
Chambersburg PA
CBHW080216040426
42333CB00044B/2704